BEING FIT

YOUR BODY IS YOUR TREASURE.

RAHEEB WAJITH

Made with ♥ on the Notion Press Platform
www.notionpress.com

Dedicated with Love to my Parents Suraiya and Abdul Wajith,

To my son Adil Rashid and niece Alisha.

To the Almighty for gifting me this wonderful life of purpose and

Finally Dear Reader Thank you ! for picking this book.

Thank you!!

Contents

Contents

Foreword

Your Body is Your Treasure, Maintain it.

Congratulations to you, you've taken the first step towards wellness. This book will teach you about fitness irrespective of your age and physical condition. Do consult a physician before you start any exercise all of a sudden.

Preface

Your body is your treasure, the perfect body adds years to life and life to years . To enjoy all the earthly pleasures it is mandatory for us to have a healthy body.If you have a healthy body you can achieve anything in this world,Nothing is impossible and you can live a life you are proud of.

The way to go is to achieve something great and that is not the end but to enjoy the privileges which comes along with the greatness for that a healthy body is the requirement. A strong and healthy body gives you a perfect feeling,a strong intuition you can achieve anything in this world.

At the same time if ***Health is lost All Is Lost*** we realise this truth only when we are sick.

"A strong mind in a strong body" Everyone deserves to be fit and strong no matter the age,

Just think how much we suffer when we get cold. It's very irritating isn't it, But usually cold disappears within a week but if some serious disease affects us like diabetes ,cancer ,heart attack and stroke, etc.., you are almost done that is why our forefathers rightly said *Health is Wealth* .

Anybook read and not put into action almost equal to the book not read so I would advise you to get into action whatever you you learn from this book ,without doing physical workout and only reading this book will take you nowhere ,There are two primary conditions for you to keep your body healthy and strong ,the the first is to aspire for a healthy body the second is the action ie. physical workouts

I repeat this: All *of us want to live young but we but not all are willing to put the effort. Small* changes in your day to day life including healthy habits and physical exercise can go a long way in maintaining your overall wellness .

Prologue

I am not a natural born athlete but boy I wish I was .

Right from my school and college I have been surrounded by people who effortlessly accomplished physical feats of dramatic strength, endurance and agility.To top it all they hardly ever seemed to workout but all of us are not not born with the same gift including me .

Over the years I have spent too much on training and discovering new methods to get lean and strong, sometimes I found myself in wrong ways I would train and train but never would change the way I look but that didn't stop me from training in fact I was determined to find the best technique to work for my body and all those knowledge I had discovered over the years of utter hard work I will share with you in this book .

I now train no more than more than 5 days a week 30 to 40 minutes at a time I eat better I sleep better and I feel better in fact my life has changed dramatically because of this Revolutionary style of training this book will teach you all about it,

You need not be a professional bodybuilder or a seasoned athlete to start training,But regular and focused training will take your confidence to move mountains.

CHAPTER ONE

What is health

Whenever we meet our friends or relatives the first thing we ask is "How are you?" we don't ask them about their assets or liabilities .This shows how important health is .

"Who do you think are healthy?" People with gigantic figures or people who are fat with big tummy are considered strong in our society and sometimes they even ask *why are you so thin* and my mother used to ask the same question to me.It took me numerous days for me to make her understand about *fat vs strong.*

Obese people are always prone to blood pressure , heart attacks and diabetes They have a higher chance of getting sick often.

We can't say that a person who doesn't show any indications of being sick is healthy, because we don't know the internal conditions of the organs and their wear and tear.Unhealthy eating and lifestyle might surprise you all of a sudden by knocking you all over ,So better late than never

.

It is our duty to maintain our body , to start working out right from today in fact the soon you start the better it is .

CHAPTER TWO

Systems of human body

10systems constitute for the functioning of the human body they are listed below

1. Skeletal system
2. Muscular system
3. Digestive system
4.Respiratory system
5.Circulatory system
6.Excretory system
7.Nervous system
8.Endocrine system
9.Reproductive system
10.Optical & auditory system

CHAPTER THREE

Heart-Engine of our body

Our heartbeat beats roughly one lakh times per day. It can vary between 72/min beats for males and 80 beats/ minute for females and for athletes it falls around 60 beats/ minute. The main function of the heart is to pump blood to various organs of the body, So the heart forms the engine of our body if any part of our body doesn't get pure blood its function is affected.

A factor that has a significant influence on the normal resting heart is age. As a general rule children and senior citizens have a high resting rate.

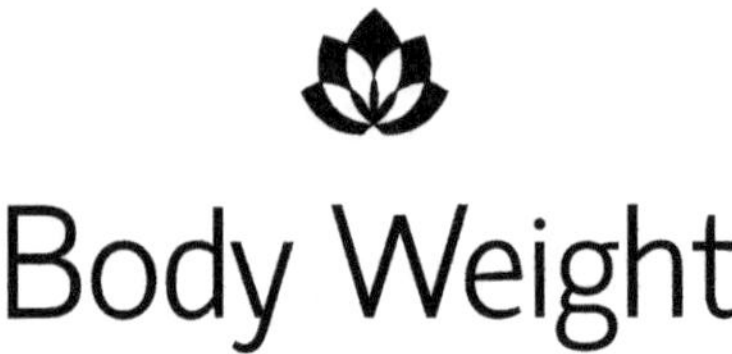

CHAPTER FOUR

Body Weight

"What is the Ideal Body Weight? "

Finding your perfect body weight does not end by looking and comparing your height and weight charts, Though it is usually considered an easy method to find the ideal body weight another factor to be determined is BMI(BODY MASS INDEX).

BMI gives you the measure of how much fat you carry on your body, It will give you a fairly accurate fat composition in the body

BMI	Considered
Below 18.5	**Underweight**
18.5 to 24.9	**Healthy Weight**
25 to 29.9	**Overweight**
30 or Higher	**Obese**

CHAPTER FIVE

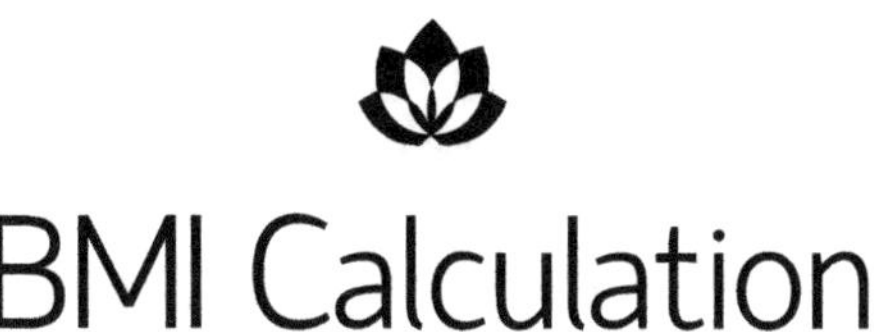

BMI Calculation

The formula for BMI was devised in the 1830s by Belgian mathematician Adolphe Quetelet and is universally expressed in kg/m^2.

BMI = weight (kg) / [height (m)]^2

Example

For an adult with height of 170 cm and weight of 65 kg.

BMI=65/(1.7)^2

BMI=65/2.89==**22.5(Healthy BMI)**

CHAPTER SIX

Blood sugar

Blood sugar is the amount of glucose present in the blood. We get glucose from the food we eat, It is vital for the functioning of various organs as it is a supply of energy and nutrients to the organs.

The absorption and production of glucose are constantly regulated by the small intestine, liver, and pancreas.

Pancreas controls the excess glucose amount in our body by secreting a hormone called insulin. The insulin sends excess glucose into the liver as glycogen.

The pancreas also produces a hormone called glucagon, which does the opposite of insulin, raising blood sugar levels when needed, the two hormones work together to keep glucose balanced. When this balance of glucose is not maintained in the blood for a long time then it causes Diabetes where our body fails to produce insulin to absorb glucose from food.

It can take decades to diagnose high blood sugar levels, But with proper exercise and diet, you can avoid it, and those who have diabetes can reduce its effect and bring it back to normal.

Normal Blood sugar levels

Before Food 80-99 mg/dl

After Food 80-140mg/dl

CHAPTER SEVEN

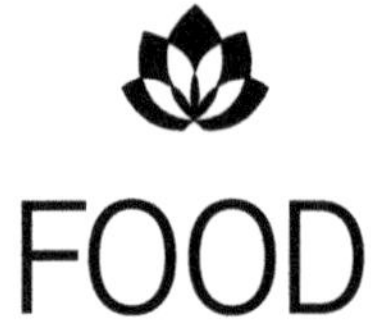

FOOD

"Let food be thy medicine and medicine be thy food."

— Hippocrates

What you eat has profound effects on your overall health.

Thus, many people argue that food is medicine.

Many illnesses can be prevented, treated, or even cured by eating the right food.

Hippocrates said almost 2500 years ago "Leave your drugs in the chemist's pot if you can heal the patient with food."

Centuries ago the earliest known physicians and health practitioners across the world imparted the benefits of using food as medicine to heal the body

Often that illness stems from inadequate nutrition and bad eating habits and if people were to learn good eating habits then their ideal health would be restored. Even before medicines were found tribal elders would seek out healing herbs and plants for their community and food would be applied prescriptively to bring about healing. Slowly through the years, man has moved away from the healing power of nature and towards synthetic and chemical compounds to cure illness.

The fact is that because we have moved away from natural remedies and rely on a diet of processed, fatty and sugar-laden food the consequences are that rates of obesity and disease have increased day by day

If food has the power to prevent many of the illnesses we experience today then it is wise to change our eating habits to use it to our own advantage to heal and prevent illness. Although taking pharma medicines may be useful in the long run they have numerous side effects and contribute to the formation of toxins in our bodies.

While Pharma medicines are important in life-threatening situations, if long-term conditions can be managed with diet and lifestyle changes then using food as medicine is the best way of tackling the issue and preventing future health problems.

There are many factors that contribute to bringing about diseases such as stress, nutrition, hormone balance, and the importance of detoxification and food.

The good news is that these can be reversed with the help of eating healthy food.

Being healthy means putting the right fuel into your body and having your inner engine function smoothly. Every meal you take should be considered this way, So that you feel the more nutritious foods you choose the healthier you will be.

Eating whole foods acts as medicine to heal and protect your body and give the immune system a break from dealing with toxins, If you are eating junk food your body will not be receiving all of the nutrients it needs to function properly.

Numerous foods have specific healing effects and do not rely on synthetic supplements which are hazardous.

Fuelling up on superfoods is a great way to provide the body with nutrients and not overeat. Individual foods have their own unique set of nutrients to meet the needs of your body so eating a wide variety of foods ensures that you are getting a diverse range of nutrients, vitamins, and minerals that you need.

Incorporating the seasons into your menu planning will benefit you so that you can enjoy fresh and in-the-moment foods that are abundantly available. There is also a cost saving when you buy in season. Shop at local growers' markets or co-ops and talk to the sellers about what's in season.

When it comes to buying healthily the best way to shop is to think about where the food you are buying actually came from, is it traceable, fresh, and at its best? Or is it housed beneath layers of packaging? Even though it takes a little longer when shopping, get used to reading labels and finding out exactly what is in the food. If it has more than six ingredients it's probably not going to be that good for you.

Shop in season and choose foods that are as close to their natural state as possible. Remember that your body will love you for it!

CHAPTER EIGHT

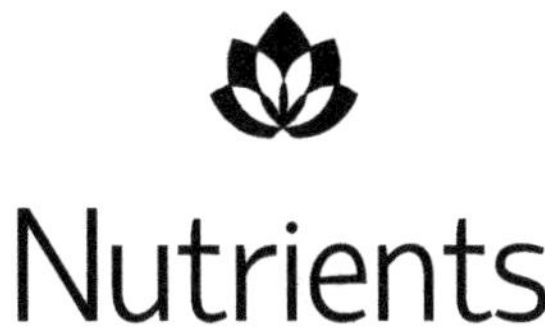

Nutrients

Many nutrients in food promote health and protect your body from disease.

Eating whole, nutritious foods is important because their unique substances work synergistically to create an effect that can't be replicated by taking a supplement.

Vitamins and minerals

Vitamins and minerals are vital for your health , deficiencies can substantially increase your risk of disease due to immune dysfunction and increase your risk of certain cancers

Nutritious foods, including fruits, vegetables, and spinach have various vitamins and minerals required for our bodies. They are filled with antioxidants.

Antioxidants protect cells from damage that may otherwise lead to disease,

Fiber

Fiber is an essential part of a healthy diet. It promotes proper digestion by feeding beneficial bacteria in your gut.

Eating vegetables, beans, grains, and fruits helps protect against disease, decrease inflammation, and boost your immune system as these are rich in fiber

Low fiber -can cause risk of illnesses, including colon cancer and stroke

Protein and healthy fats

Protein is an essential nutrient to keep your body functioning well. Proteins are part of every cell in your body and are needed to build and repair muscle, tissue, skin, nails, and hair. Protein also helps build hormones and enzymes. They are the building blocks of our body

Protein helps in muscle synthesis, metabolism, and growth.

Here are some tips for healthy protein choices.

Mostly protein

Meat, poultry, fish, eggs, tofu

Some protein

Legumes, nuts, nut butters, seeds, seed butters, milk, cheese, cottage cheese, soy beverages, yogurt

Little protein

Whole grain breads, rice, pasta, quinoa, barley

How much protein is required

1 gram of protein is required per kg body weight.ie If you are 60 kg then you need 60 g of protein.

Bodybuilders, Athletes, and martial artists will take upto 2gram of protein per kg of body weight.

There are many vegetarian sources of protein. Eggs, low-fat cheese, yogurt, and milk are good animal protein sources. Vegans can enjoy beans, lentils, dried peas, tofu, nuts, and seeds. Vegetables and grain products all contain small amounts of protein too.

Carbohydrates

Carbohydrates provide the energy required for the body to perform its day-to-day tasks. Our diet should be filled with 60% of carbs

.Common sources of naturally occurring carbohydrates include: Rice, Wheat Fruit, Vegetables, Legumes, Nuts, and Grains

Types of carbohydrates

There are three main types of carbohydrates:

· **Sugar.** Sugar is the simplest form of carbohydrate and occurs naturally in some foods, including fruits, vegetables, milk, and milk products. Types of sugar include fruit sugar (fructose), table sugar (sucrose), and milk sugar (lactose).

· **Starch.** Starch is a complex carbohydrate, meaning it is made of many sugar units bonded together. Starch occurs naturally in vegetables, grains, and cooked dry beans and peas.

· **Fiber.** Fiber also is a complex carbohydrate. It occurs naturally in fruits, vegetables, whole grains, and cooked dry beans and peas.

· Terms such as "low carb" or "net carbs" often appear on product labels. But the Food and Drug Administration doesn’t regulate these terms, so there’s no standard meaning. Typically "net carbs" is used to mean the number of carbohydrates in a product excluding fiber or excluding both fiber and sugar alcohols.

You probably have also heard talk about the glycemic index. The glycemic index classifies carbohydrate-containing foods according to their potential to raise your blood sugar level.

Weight-loss diets based on the glycemic index typically recommend limiting foods that are higher on the glycemic index. Foods with a relatively high glycemic index ranking include potatoes and white bread, and less healthy options such as snack foods and desserts that contain refined flours.

Many healthy foods, such as whole grains, legumes, vegetables, fruits, and low-fat dairy products, are naturally lower on the glycemic index.

How much carbohydrates do you need?

Carbohydrates make up 45 to 65 percent of your total daily calories.

So, if you get 2,000 calories a day, between 900 and 1,300 calories should be from carbohydrates. That translates to between 225 and 325 grams of carbohydrates a day.

You can find the carbohydrate content of packaged foods on the Nutrition Facts label. The label shows total carbohydrates — which includes starches, fiber, sugar alcohols, and naturally occurring and added sugars. The label might also list separately total fiber, soluble fiber and sugar.

.

Carbohydrates and your health

Despite their bad rap, carbohydrates are vital to your health for a number of reasons.

Providing energy

Carbohydrates are your body's main fuel source. During digestion, sugars and starches are broken down into simple sugars. They're then absorbed into your bloodstream, where they're known as blood sugar (blood glucose).

From there, glucose enters your body's cells with the help of insulin. Glucose is used by your body for energy, and fuels all of your activities — whether it's going for a jog or simply breathing. Extra glucose is stored in your liver, muscles, and other cells for later use, or is converted to fat.

Protecting against disease

Some evidence suggests that whole grains and dietary fiber from whole foods help reduce your risk of cardiovascular diseases. Fiber may also protect against obesity and type 2 diabetes. Fiber is also essential for optimal digestive health.

Controlling weight

Evidence shows that eating plenty of fruit, vegetables, and whole grains can help you control your weight. Their bulk and fiber content aids weight control by helping you feel full on fewer calories. Contrary to what low-carb diets claim, very few studies show that a diet rich in healthy carbohydrates leads to weight gain or obesity.

Choose your carbohydrates wisely

Carbohydrates are an essential part of a healthy diet and provide many important nutrients. Still, not all carbs are created equal.

Aim for whole fresh, frozen, and canned fruits and vegetables without added sugar. Other options are fruit juices and dried fruits. Whole fruits and vegetables also add fiber.

whole grains. Whole grains are better sources than refined grains of fiber and other important nutrients, such as B vitamins. Refined grains go through a process that strips out parts of the grain — along with some of the nutrients and fiber.

· **low-fat dairy products.** Milk, cheese, yogurt, and other dairy products are good sources of calcium and protein, plus many other vitamins and minerals. Consider the low-fat versions, to help limit calories and saturated fat. And beware of dairy products that have added sugar.

legumes. Legumes — which include beans, peas, and lentils — are among the most versatile and nutritious foods available. They are typically low in fat and high in folate, potassium, iron, and magnesium..

CHAPTER NINE

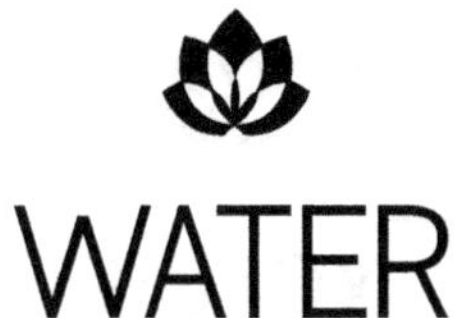

WATER

Getting enough water every day is important for your health. Healthy people meet their needs by drinking water when. Most of your fluid needs are met through water since our body constitutes roughly 72% water. Water maintains your body temperature and gets rid of wastes through urination, perspiration, and bowel movements,

Roughly drinking 1.6 liters of water can be good for your health. Drinking too much water leads to a loss in sodium levels so don't overdrink it or under drink it,

Research tells us that people who drink water on an empty stomach are less prone to disease.

So start drinking anywhere between 0.5l to 1l once you wake up on empty stomach. This can also help with weight management

CHAPTER TEN

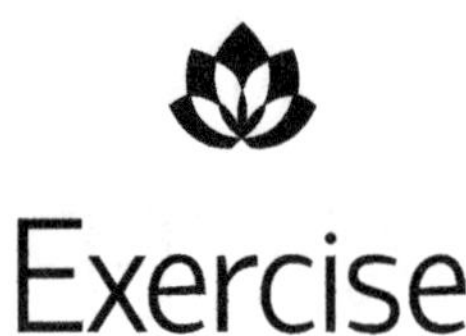

Exercise

Exercise does your mind and body a world of goodness instantly. The moment you start to run, launch into your spin class, or start your Pilates session, the benefits would start to kick in. "We see changes in the body within seconds," Your heart rate increases and blood is delivered to your muscles. You feel the blood pump adrenaline rush,and fat burn after an intense workout

As little as 30 minutes per day to five days a week is what it takes to increase your well being.

.When you do cardio your brain sends signals to lungs to help you breathe faster and deeper, delivering extra oxygen to your muscles.

.

Benefits of Exercise...

Exercise elevates your level of immunoglobulins, which are proteins that help improve the immune system and ward off infection. Mood-enhancing chemicals, like serotonin, dopamine, and norepinephrine, flood your brain for a couple of hours post-exercise.You're adding lean muscle your muscles are now starting to rebuild themselves and repair the microscopic tears that come with lifting weights, or pushing your body against gravity

Your heart is healthier. One of the major benefits of working out can be found in how your heart functions. One sweat session lowers your blood pressure for up to 16 hours

You're a quick study. You're super alert and focused post-exercise. That's because a good workout increases the flow of blood and oxygen to your brain

You're feeling zen. This benefits of working out lasts for up to a day if competed in a marathon event like a marathon. Stress? What stress?

You're blasting more calories, even at rest. "For every 100 calories you burn during your workout, you can expect to burn 15 calories after,". If you went on a five-km run, you would torch about 300 calories, which could mean zapping an extra 45 later.

You're hungry. Now that you've burned through your energy stores, your blood sugar levels are dropping. Just how low they go depends on how much you ate or drank before your workout and how long and intensely you exercised.

You're adding years to your life. Fitness buffs have better telomeres, the DNA that bookends our chromosomes and protects them from damage, which can slow the aging process.

You feel fantastic. Just four months of exercise is as good as prescription meds at boosting mood and reducing depression. Keep it up and not only will your life be longer, it will be happier, too!

CHAPTER ELEVEN

How to Get an Effective Working Out

As if all those benefits of working out weren't enough, we scored a few bonus tips from the pros for how to turn up the volume even more.

1. **Strength training twice a week or more.** It will Supercharge your metabolism so that you'll continue to burn calories for longer. Make the most of this benefit of working out by turning up the intensity of your workouts to burn more fat and calories. Raise the incline on the treadmill, run up stairs or hills, crank the resistance on your cycle.

2. **Do fewer crunches and more planks.** Begin on all fours, hands under shoulders, knees under hips, then lower forearms to floor and extend legs straight behind you, balancing on toes. Keeping abs engaged and back flat, hold for 30 seconds; do 10 reps three or four times a week. Limit crunches to no more than three sets of 15 at a time. Anything beyond that isn't doing you much good.

3. **Try HIIT (or other interval-style workouts).** You may feel even happier. People who do interval training

experience a bigger boost in mood immediately following their workout than those who exercise at a steady pace, Olson says.

CHAPTER TWELVE

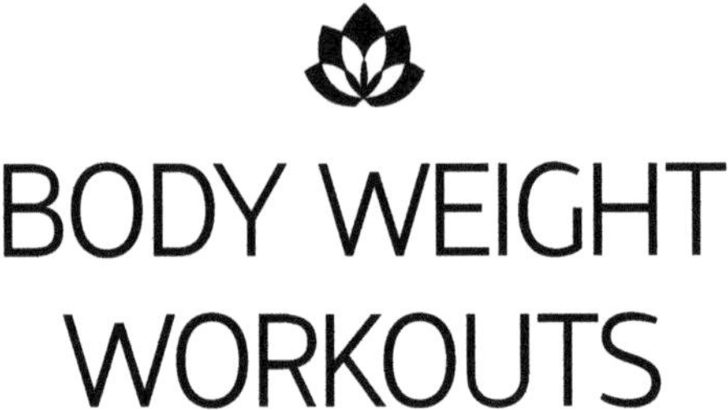

BODY WEIGHT WORKOUTS

The main advantage of body weight workouts aka calisthenics is they can be performed anywhere anytime without any equipments ,They build the raw strength ,by pushing our body against gravity by varying resistance tensions are caused in tendons and muscle fibers which makes us so strong ,Imagine Cave man's strength vs Today's bodybuilders

If you're planning on following a calisthenics workout program, you should be prepared for full body workouts.

Most bodybuilding workouts typically focus on isolation exercises, working one specific muscle region per day.

With calisthenics and bodyweight workouts, **that's impossible to do**. Most calisthenics exercises are **compound exercises**, which means that **they target several muscle groups at the same time.**

For example: A chin-up targets your back, shoulders and biceps. While dumbbell curls only target the bicep.

Full body workouts

Full Body Bodyweight Workouts composed of only compound movements bring many benefits such as:

They're a more natural form of training

If you're a beginner, it's normal that you have some form of muscular imbalances, the most common being the dominant arm being much stronger than the other. It may also happen if you've been training for a few months or years using only isolation exercises using poor form following bad routines. In order to keep this from happening, committing to full-body workout routines is one of the best things you can do. This will make it very hard for you to have muscular imbalances because you'll have to work all the targeted muscles with the same intensity

They Save Time

Full Body Workout routines are typically split into 3 days during the week. For Example Monday, Wednesday, and Friday. The rest days in between are essential so that your muscles have time to recover and grow from the tough workout you just gave them.

This means that you have two/three free days for your other daily tasks or cardio sessions.

With isolation routines, you usually have to work out **5 days a week** so that you can target all the desired muscles in your body and maintain proper muscle balance.

Workout "Skip Ability"

This can be both a negative and a positive point.

On one hand, full-body workouts are great for a busy person because if you have no other choice than to skip a workout, there's no harm in skipping it and sometimes it's even beneficial to add an extra rest day. Unlike isolation-based workouts where it's crucial that you complete every workout of the week otherwise you risk having muscular imbalances.

But on the other hand, this workout "skip ability" may lead to laziness and it'll give you extra excuses to skip a workout.

Faster Workouts

Compound exercises can be super intense. You'll be training so many parts of your body in such a low time interval that you'll be completely wrecked in no time. And with the increased heart rate and intensity and some super sets in between, your workouts will also be a form of cardio, saving you loads of time.

Now that I've convinced you to start doing full body workouts, here's one battle-tested calisthenics full body workout you should try today.

CHAPTER THIRTEEN

Exercise routine

Here is a calisthenics workout for beginners that works various parts of the body for a complete, full-body workout:

Perform the following exercise circuit three times, with a 30-second rest between each exercise set, and a three-minute rest between each circuit repetition.

10 pull-ups

1. Stand facing an exercise bar.
2. Grasp the bar from the top with your arms slightly more than shoulder-width apart.
3. Use your shoulder muscles to pull you up, bringing your head up over the bar.

10 chin-ups

1. Stand facing an exercise bar.
2. Grasp the bar from underneath with your arms in a tight, slightly closer than shoulder-width grip.

1. Use your biceps to pull you up, bringing your head up over the bar.

20 dips

1. Stand inside a dip bar and use your arms and shoulders to lift yourself off the ground.

2. Bend your elbows back using your tricep muscles to move you up and down.

If you do not have a dip bar, you can also perform dips off an exercise ball or bench by keeping your feet on the ground and knees bent at a 90-degree angle.

25 jump squats

1. Stand with your body facing forward and your feet parallel, directly underneath your shoulders.

2. Move your feet a few inches apart with your toes pointed slightly outward.

3. Lower yourself into the squat, lowering your hips back and down while bending your knees.

4. Keep your chest upright, with your head and face forward.

5. Get into as deep a squat as possible, and then explode forcefully upward into a jump.

Never extend your knees over your toes, as that moves the strain of the squat to the knee joints. This can injure your knee joints.

20 pushups

1. Get on your knees and place your hands underneath, but slightly outside, your shoulders.

2. Extend your legs while holding your body up with your arms, getting into the "plank" position.

3. Be careful not to let your back sag or backside stick up into the air.

4. Lower your body by bending your elbows close to your body until your chest almost touches the floor.

5. Your upper arms should form a 45-degree angle when the top part of your body is in the lower pushup position.

6. Pause while you are in the lower position, and then push back up to the starting position quickly.

7. Keep your abdomen, or core, flexed during the entire movement.

50 crunches

1. Lay on the ground with your back flat.

2. Place your feet flat on the ground, bending your knees up at a 90-degree angle to your body.

3. Cross your hands on top of your chest and keep your head about a fist's distance from your chest.

4. Keeping your core tight, sit up until your elbows or chest touch your knees.

5. Focus on using your core muscles to pull you up, breathing out as you sit up and breathing in as you lie down.

Burpees 10

1. Stand facing forward with your feet shoulder-width apart, keeping your weight in your heels and your arms at your sides.

2. Push your hips back, bending your knees and lowering into a squat.

3. Put your hands palms down on the floor in front of you, a little narrower than you are keeping your feet.

4. Put your weight into your hands and jump your feet back, landing softly on the balls of your feet, your body in a straight plank position.

5. Be careful not to let your back sag or backside stick up into the air.

6. Jump your feet forward so they land next to your hands.

7. Push your arms up over your head and jump quickly into the air.

30 seconds of jump rope

1. Grasp the jump rope handles and hold your hands roughly the same distance from the centerline of your body.

2. Rotate the rope with your wrists — not your elbows or shoulders — while jumping off the ground about one to two inches into the air, clearing the rope.

3. As you jump, keep your toes pointed down and a slight bend in your knees.

The takeaway

Calisthenics exercises appear to increase physical fitness to a similar degree as weight-based training exercises. The benefit of calisthenics over weight-based training exercises is that calisthenics requires little-to-no additional equipment — all you need is your body!

CHAPTER FOURTEEN

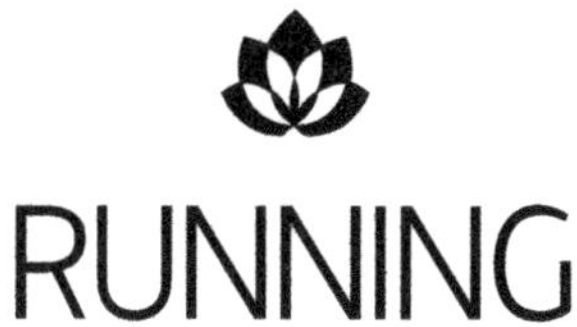

RUNNING

"Running-King of all exercise" -Bruce lee

Think you don't have time to train today? Think again. Research shows that just 30 minutes of running can have huge benefits on your short-term and long-term health. Here are the top reasons to lace up your shoes and squeeze in that run today.

Burn FatRunning for just 15-30 minutes will kick-start your metabolism and burn some serious fat, both during and after the exercise itself. That's because, during a shorter run, your body will use fat as its primary power source, rather than relying on the carbohydrates that play a bigger role as exercise intensity increases.

You'll also keep burning fat long after your run. After intense physical activity, your body goes into EPOC mode (excess post-exercise oxygen consumption), where it uses the energy from fat and carbohydrates to restore itself to its pre-exercise state. EPOC can last from 15 minutes to a whopping 48 hours; so that 30-minute run could keep you burning fat for 2 whole days.

Simply put, running makes you feel good – even if you can't do it for that long. Just 10 minutes of aerobic exercise releases a large amount of the mood-boosting endorphins responsible for "runner's high," so a quick lunchtime run can make you feel just as good as a longer one. The benefits aren't just in the moment, either; regular running has countless long-term effects on your mental health, from decreased stress and anxiety to improved energy levels. If you don't trust the research, just try out short, regular runs for a month and see the effects yourself.

If you keep your run to 30 minutes, you're very unlikely to overstretch or overuse your muscles. **That means a much lower risk of injury.** As long as you take the usual stretching and cool-down measures to recover properly, your body will feel readier and more refreshed when it comes to your next long run. Even if you usually go for longer distances, factoring in the occasional 30-minute run as part of your regular exercise routine can be much better for your body in the long term.

One 30-minute run is guaranteed to burn between 200-500 calories. That's a fantastic step forward to your weight loss goal. Or a guilt-free guilty pleasure that day. Or splitting the bottle instead of having a glass. Whatever your goals and priorities are, calorie wiggle room is always good news.

When you start running regularly for 30 minutes, **you'll see your sleep improve significantly.** And even if you're used to more strenuous exercise, a shorter run will still give you better sleep than no running at all.

That's true for both quality and quantity: you'll both fall asleep faster and spend more time in those deep sleep stages which are crucial for physical recovery. There's a caveat to this though: try not to schedule your run before bedtime. All those feel-good endorphins will also make you feel alert and awake, so you may struggle to get to sleep in the first place.

If you can run 3-5 days a week for 30 minutes, the internal health benefits will very quickly start to show on the surface, too. **You'll soon see effects like more defined muscles, pounds off the scale, and clearer healthy skin your** muscles will be stronger so you can get more out of those gym sessions, and your improved cardio fitness will allow you to try things you perhaps couldn't before. And that means more confidence, too.

It's a big claim, but the studies show it's true. **The fitness level you achieve from regular, shorter runs can add life to your years** There are a ton of reasons for this: improved circulation, lower blood pressure, a better balance of good and bad cholesterol, lower stress hormones. Your quality of life will also be higher; a basic level of fitness has been linked consistently to better brain and memory function in later years.

The bottom line is that even when you think you don't have that much time, there's no excuse not to get out for a quick 30 minute run

CHAPTER FIFTEEN

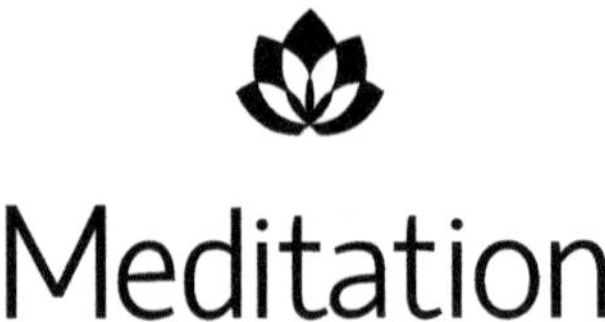

Meditation

Meditation can wipe away the day's stress, bringing with it inner peace. See how you can easily learn to practice meditation whenever you need it most.

If stress has you anxious, tense and worried, consider trying meditation. Spending even a few minutes in meditation can restore your calm and inner peace.

Anyone can practice meditation. It's simple and inexpensive, and it doesn't require any special equipment.

And you can practice meditation wherever you are — whether you're out for a walk, riding the bus, waiting at the doctor's office or even in the middle of a difficult business meeting.

Understanding meditation

Meditation has been practiced for thousands of years. Meditation originally was meant to help deepen understanding of the sacred and mystical forces of life. These days, meditation is commonly used for relaxation and stress reduction.

Meditation is considered a type of mind-body complementary medicine. Meditation can produce a deep state of relaxation and a tranquil mind.

During meditation, you focus your attention and eliminate the stream of jumbled thoughts that may be crowding your mind and causing stress. This process may result in enhanced physical and emotional well-being.

Benefits of meditation

Meditation can give you a sense of calm, peace and balance that can benefit both your emotional well-being and your overall health.

And these benefits don't end when your meditation session ends. Meditation can help carry you more calmly through your day and may help you manage symptoms of certain medical conditions.

Meditation and emotional well-being

When you meditate, you may clear away the information overload that builds up every day and contributes to your stress.

The emotional benefits of meditation can include:

· Gaining a new perspective on stressful situations
· Building skills to manage your stress
· Increasing self-awareness
· Focusing on the present
· Reducing negative emotions
· Increasing imagination and creativity
· Increasing patience and tolerance

Meditation and illness

Meditation might also be useful if you have a medical condition, especially one that may be worsened by stress.

While a growing body of scientific research supports the health benefits of meditation, some researchers believe it's not yet possible to draw conclusions about the possible benefits of meditation.

With that in mind, some research suggests that meditation may help people manage symptoms of conditions such as:

- Anxiety
- Asthma
- Cancer
- Chronic pain
- Depression
- Heart disease
- High blood pressure
- Irritable bowel syndrome
- Sleep problems
- Tension headaches

Be sure to talk to your health care provider about the pros and cons of using meditation if you have any of these conditions or other health problems. In some cases, meditation can worsen symptoms associated with certain mental and physical health conditions.

Meditation isn't a replacement for traditional medical treatment. But it may be a useful addition to your other treatment.

Elements of meditation

Different types of meditation may include different features to help you meditate. These may vary depending on whose guidance you follow or who's teaching a class. Some of the most common features in meditation include:

· **Focused attention.** Focusing your attention is generally one of the most important elements of meditation.

Focusing your attention is what helps free your mind from the many distractions that cause stress and worry. You can focus your attention on such things as a specific object, an image, a mantra, or even your breathing.

· **Relaxed breathing.** This technique involves deep, even-paced breathing using the diaphragm muscle to expand your lungs. The purpose is to slow your breathing, take in more oxygen, and reduce the use of shoulder, neck and upper chest muscles while breathing so that you breathe more efficiently.

· **A quiet setting.** If you're a beginner, practicing meditation may be easier if you're in a quiet spot with few distractions, including no television, radios or cellphones.

As you get more skilled at meditation, you may be able to do it anywhere, especially in high-stress situations where you benefit the most from meditation, such as a traffic jam, a stressful work meeting or a long line at the grocery store.

· **A comfortable position.** You can practice meditation whether you're sitting, lying down, walking, or in other positions or activities. Just try to be comfortable so that you can get the most out of your meditation. Aim to keep good posture during meditation.

· **Open attitude.** Let thoughts pass through your mind without judgment.

Everyday ways to practice meditation

Don't let the thought of meditating the "right" way add to your stress. If you choose to, you can attend special meditation centers or group classes led by trained instructors. But you can also practice meditation easily on your own.

And you can make meditation as formal or informal as you like, however it suits your lifestyle and situation. Some people build meditation into their daily routine. For example, they may start and end each day with an hour of meditation. But all you really need is a few minutes of quality time for meditation.

Here are some ways you can practice meditation on your own, whenever you choose:

· **Breathe deeply.** This technique is good for beginners because breathing is a natural function.

Focus all your attention on your breathing. Concentrate on feeling and listening as you inhale and exhale through your nostrils. Breathe deeply and slowly. When your attention wanders, gently return your focus to your breathing.

· **Scan your body.** When using this technique, focus attention on different parts of your body. Become aware of your body's various sensations, whether that's pain, tension, warmth or relaxation.

Combine body scanning with breathing exercises and imagine breathing heat or relaxation into and out of different parts of your body..

· **Walk and meditate.** Combining a walk with meditation is an efficient and healthy way to relax. You can use this technique anywhere you're walking, such as in a tranquil forest, on a city sidewalk or at the mall.

When you use this method, slow down your walking pace so that you can focus on each movement of your legs or feet. Don't focus on a particular destination. Concentrate on your legs and feet, repeating action words in your mind such as "lifting," "moving" and "placing" as you lift each foot, move your leg forward and place your foot on the ground.

· **Engage in prayer.** Prayer is the best known and most widely practiced example of meditation. Spoken and written prayers are found in most faith traditions.

You can pray using your own words or read prayers written by others. Check the self-help section of your local bookstore for examples. Talk with your rabbi, priest, pastor or other spiritual leader about possible resources.

· **Read and reflect.** Many people report that they benefit from reading poems or sacred texts, and taking a few moments to quietly reflect on their meaning.

You can also listen to sacred music, spoken words, or any music you find relaxing or inspiring. You may want to write your reflections in a journal or discuss them with a friend or spiritual leader.

· **Focus on your love and gratitude.** In this type of meditation, you focus your attention on a sacred image or being, weaving feelings of love, compassion and gratitude into your thoughts. You can also close your eyes and use your imagination or gaze at representations of the image.

Don't judge your meditation skills, which may only increase your stress. Meditation takes practice.

Keep in mind, for instance, that it's common for your mind to wander during meditation, no matter how long you've been practicing meditation. If you're meditating to calm your mind and your attention wanders, slowly return to the object, sensation or movement you're focusing on.

Experiment, and you'll likely find out what types of meditation work best for you and what you enjoy doing. Adapt meditation to your needs at the moment. Remember, there's no right way or wrong way to meditate. What matters is that meditation helps you reduce your stress and feel better overall.

CHAPTER SIXTEEN

No time to Exercise

"Did you exercise today?"

"No, I didn't have time?"

That's the most common answer given when asked *why people don't exercise* regularly. Nobody has enough time. Guess what?

People don't skip out on exercise because they don't think it's good for them. People don't exercise because they'd rather be doing something else.

Let's deal with this problem.

"Whats the reason?"

I would share you a recent study I came across recently came across that discussed how people are spending their time these days:

· The average man spends 8 hours/day working while women spend 7.1 hours

· Both sexes spend almost **an hour commuting** to and from work!

· Women do a greater share of housework (2.8 hours per day vs. 2.1 for men)

· Men spend more time doing leisure activities (5.4 hours vs. 4.8)

· **TV is still the leisure activity of choice** (taking up almost 1/2 of the leisure time)

· The Internet is catching up -It accounts for almost 2 hours per day!

· In one month the average person spends **15 hours on social media!**

Don't lie to yourself – You DO have time to get up and move!

So, do you really ever have "no time" for exercise? Of course not. You can always find time to do exercise, but only if it's a priority. Let's just be honest here – Checking your Mobile news feed is often more important/valuable/enjoyable than exercising. The stats are very clear that this is true.

Knowing this certainly doesn't solve the problem though (it might just make us all feel guilty for spending so much time in front of the TV or computer!). What's next?...

CHAPTER SEVENTEEN

The Solution

The root cause of our sedentary lifestyles is not a lack of time. We have time to exercise but we don't do it– that's the problem we need to solve. Here is a simple and effective 3-step process that can help you permanently change the way you think about exercise AND how it fits into your life:

Identify The REAL Problem

It's NOT a problem if you don't go to the gym, don't run, don't bike anywhere, or don't do hot yoga. **It IS a problem if you don't move your body.**

A research compilation by the World Health Organization concluded that 9% of all premature deaths are directly caused by inactivity. We are killing ourselves because we don't get up and move our bodies each and every day.

A lack of movement is the real problem, not a lack of exercise. Exercise sounds like something that only fit people do, but moving is something for everyone.

You do not have to kill yourself during exercise in order to enjoy the health benefits that come with being active.

The researchers found that the **intense exercisers felt "deserving" after their longer workouts** and would end up eating much more than the light exercise group members. In contrast, the **light exercisers became motivated** by their small doses of exercise and became even more active throughout their day (e.g. choosing to take the stairs instead of the elevator).

In step #1 we identified that *movement* is what your body needs. The term "exercise" might conjure up images of high-intensity bootcamp classes, endless running on a treadmill, or playing some sort of competitive **sport.** These are all great BUT they are not the solution to the exercise problem for most people.

If you are not physically active each day then it's time to re-frame what exercise might look like for you. Finding any way to move your body can have exceptional health benefits, maybe even more so than intense exercise will provide.

Make One Small Change Today

Recap: Everyone knows exercise is "healthy" but many people say they *don't have time* really because they don't *want* to do it. In many cases, people don't want to "exercise" because they think it has to be physically exhausting in order to be effective. This is a lie. What everyone really needs (yes, you!) is daily movement.

What are you going to do about it?

Most people quit before they even start because the process of change seems too daunting. It

I'm all about **action steps**. If you aren't moving your body each and every day then I encourage you to follow these actions steps beginning today:

Start Small – Even 10 minutes per day is better than not exercising at all. Set a daily exercise goal that is 100% achievable for the next 2 weeks. If you make it happen then you can re-evaluate that goal for the following 2 weeks (choose something that is again 100% achievable). Soon you won't even be able to remember life without exercise daily movement.

· **Get Accountable** – Nobody should start alone. It's too easy to cheat, to fall behind, or to stop altogether if you don't have someone holding you accountable. Find a friend who might want to start exercising with you, post your goal on Facebook, or at least tell someone about what you plan to do. Simply saying a goal aloud makes it real and much more likely to achieve and doing it with a friend is even better.

How do you plan to get your daily dose of movement? Tell someone (or lots of people!)

· **Plan It Out** – Change rarely happens without a plan. When can you best schedule exercise into your day? Picking a regular time is the best way to make exercise a permanent addition to your schedule. Telling yourself that you will “squeeze it in somewhere” just leaves the door open for other items to crop up and push exercise to the bottom of the priority list.

What Are You Upto?

If you're not "exercising" each day because you're too busy then you are telling a lie and you are sacrificing your health and longevity. Exercise is not what many people think it is – It doesn't have to be sweaty, or painful, or exhausting. It does require movement and it is something that you can do every day.

One Last Request

If you have enjoyed reading this book please be kind enough to add review for it, as it will be helpful for me to upgrade this book and also my future writing career,Reviews are the lifeblood of any books on amazon and especially for independent authors ,If you would click 5 stars on kindle reading device that will ensure that i will continue to write more books.A quick rating or review helps me to support my family and I deeply appreciate it,Without stars you wouldn't have found this book.Please take 10 second of your time to support an independent author like me

9 798889 758464

Printed by Libri Plureos GmbH in Hamburg, Germany